POWER OF UBIQUINOL

THE KEY TO **ENERGY, VITALITY**, AND A **HEALTHY HEART**

ROBERT BARRY, PH.D.

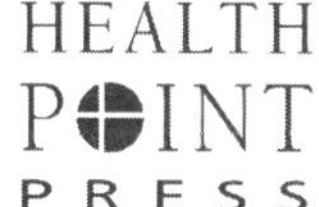

Cover design: Jeannie Tudor
Editor: Lisa Kaspin
Book design and typesetting: Gary A. Rosenberg

Health Point Press
4335 Van Nuys Blvd.
Sherman Oaks, CA 91403
818-788-2040

ISBN: 0-9774356-5-2

Printed in the United States of America.

10   9   8   7   6   5   4   3   2   1

Contents

Introduction

In this updated edition of *The Power of Ubiquinol*, we focus on the latest research on the benefits of Ubiquinol. In particular, we describe its ability to improve the health of patients with cardio-vascular disease.

More and more attention is being devoted to the prevention of diseases commonly associated with aging. Though diet and exercise can play a role in prevention of such diseases and cardiovascular disease in particular, in recent years medical practitioners have looked to powerful compounds known as antioxidants, which neutralize free radicals in the body, thus preventing cellular damage that can contribute to these diseases.

Other aging-related concerns include less life-threatening but more immediate, quality-of-life-related, issues: fatigue and lack of stamina and energy. Approximately 20% of Americans report having fatigue intense enough to interfere with normal activities; 10%–20% of all patients who visit general practitioners complain of prolonged fatigue.[1]

To address these concerns about aging, the field of bioenergetics is receiving increased attention. Bioenergetics is defined as the study of the production and transformation of energy in cellular systems. All of our metabolic systems require constant energy input in order to function properly for continuous cellular growth, development and maintenance.

Addressing both the cellular energy and the antioxidant needs is Ubiquinol, the active antioxidant form of coenzyme Q10 (CoQ10). CoQ10 is a major component in the generation of cellular energy, and this active antioxidant form (Ubiquinol) has been described as the strongest lipid-soluble antioxidant known that is bio-synthesized in the cells. In this booklet, we define Ubiquinol, its history and ever-increasing role as a critical component for healthy aging. We will also discuss the different forms of CoQ10—the oxidized form, ubiquinone, and the reduced form, Ubiquinol—found in our bodies, define the differences between the two forms, explain who will benefit most from which form and why, and provide dosage information based on clinical evaluation.

With aging, the ability of our bodies to produce and metabolize CoQ10 declines, possibly from increased metabolic demand, diseases, insufficient dietary intake, deficiency of factors required for biosynthesis, gene mutation, and oxidative insult. Some reports state that this decline in CoQ10 becomes apparent around 40 years of age, while other reports state that it can occur as early as 20 years with slow but continuous decline. In addition and most importantly, with age and/or certain diseases or conditions, the body's ability to convert CoQ10 to its active antioxidant form, Ubiquinol, is also diminished. The result is insufficient levels of this critical active antioxidant form, in turn leading to decreases in cellular energy production and antioxidant protection. In particular, the heart requires high levels of energy, and normal heart cells contain an especially high concentration of Ubiquinol. In those with heart disease, however, the concentration of Ubiquinol and total CoQ10 is often below normal, and supplementation with the conventional CoQ10 form (ubiquinone) has not always been sufficient to improve outcomes. In this booklet, we discuss how supplementation with Ubiquinol can address the limitations of dosing with the conventional CoQ10 form. We will review the results of clinical studies evaluating the role of Ubiquinol in improving heart health. Other tips for heart-healthy living are also provided.

Finally, we will answer some of your most frequently asked questions concerning Ubiquinol.

CHAPTER 1

Aging and Quality of Life

Among the ever-increasing aging population more and more attention is being devoted to prevention and intervention, for the aging process itself along with a myriad of age-related diseases. While cardiovascular disease and neurodegenerative disease often top the list, aging also leads to more immediate issues related to everyday quality of life: increased fatigue and the lack of stamina and energy associated with aging.

In everyday life we have all experienced mild fatigue, whether due to a passing illness or a period of stress. Upon reaching middle age, we may even *expect* fatigue to accompany the aging process, acknowledging that our energy is not what it used to be when we were young. However, fatigue can be so persistent and so debilitating that it interrupts the ability to live a normal life. Ongoing fatigue for 6 months or more concurrently with symptoms such as impaired concentration, un-refreshing sleep, and muscle pain may indicate chronic fatigue syndrome (CFS). CFS affects more than one million people in the United States annually, but according to the Centers for Disease Control (CDC), tens of millions of people with similar fatiguing illness do not fully meet the strict research definition of CFS.[2] A randomized phone survey in Georgia conducted by the CDC found that 1 in 40 adults ages 18–59 met less restrictive diagnostic criteria for chronic fatigue.[3] No definitive cause for CFS has yet been identified, though recent studies suggest that the condition is linked to a genetic predisposition and may have multiple underpinnings.

For those who suffer from fatigue symptoms but do not meet the clinical definition of CFS, there are other possible causes:

- Anemia
- Use of alcohol or narcotics
- Sleep disorders
- Depression or grief
- Ongoing pain
- Underlying infection or disease
- An underactive thyroid

Since fatigue can be a hallmark of a more serious health concern, those with fatigue symptoms are advised to see their doctors.

TREATING FATIGUE

There is no known pharmaceutical cure for fatigue or CFS; medical treatment is typically aimed at relieving symptoms. Lifestyle changes, including reduction of stress and modification of diet, are usually suggested along with drug therapies to alleviate sleep problems or pain. However, since fatigue is often overlooked or dismissed by physicians, many individuals with fatigue try to self-treat in a variety of different ways, sometimes to the detriment of their health.

While stimulants like caffeine may seem like an attractive way to get a boost of energy, consuming sodas and coffee drinks may only exacerbate the fatigue and introduce a host of other problems. Caffeine stimulates the nervous system, and too much can leave you feeling restless, anxious and irritable. It can also interfere with sleep and cause headaches and abnormal heart rhythms. Furthermore, when caffeine intake is stopped, withdrawal symptoms can worsen the fatigue. If sugared sodas are your caffeine vehicle of choice, you'll also be adding unwanted calories and raising blood sugar levels, which can lead to weight gain and diabetes. Increased soft drink consumption has also been linked to osteoporosis because sodas can lower calcium levels while raising phosphate levels, resulting in calcium being pulled out of the bones.

ADDITIONAL STRATEGIES FOR PREVENTING FATIGUE

Regardless of the cause of your fatigue, you may benefit from following as many of these recommendations as possible:

- **Manage stress.** When we experience stress, our adrenal glands secrete cortisol, which prepares our bodies for "fight or flight." This is useful if we're facing down a woolly mammoth, but not so useful for everyday stresses such as traffic, relationship turmoil, and money management. Sustained high cortisol levels can lead to adrenal fatigue and a compromised immune system. Though it's difficult to avert stress entirely, consider stress-management techniques such as yoga, meditation, or other relaxation techniques.

- **Avoid overexertion.** In addition to managing stressors better, consider organizing your life to preempt as many as possible. Aim for a reasonable work and personal schedule.

- **Get enough sleep.** Cheating yourself out of a good night's rest sets the stage for fatigue the following day. On average, a person needs 8 hours of sleep per night. If you get less than this, you will be operating with a sleep debt and increased fatigue symptoms.

- **Exercise moderately.** Chronic fatigue sufferers may find it painful or difficult to exercise. Vigorous physical activity may even worsen fatigue symptoms. However, a sedentary lifestyle increases your risk for obesity and heart disease, among other health complications. Moderate exercise may increase your stamina and help you sleep better at night. Pace yourself and slowly increase the intensity. If aerobic exercise exacerbates your symptoms, try lifting light weights or doing gentle stretching.

- **Maintain a healthy diet.** Eat a balanced diet that includes plenty of lean protein, fruits and vegetables, lowfat or nonfat dairy products, and whole grains. Avoid foods high in salt and saturated fats as well as heavily processed or highly sweetened foods. The "sugar rush" you get from eating sweets sets you up for a fatigue crash; to avoid this, choose carbohydrates with a low glycemic index such as brown rice and whole wheat pastas and breads. Eat a combination of protein and carbohydrates at each meal, especially lunch, for optimal alertness. Consume foods rich in iron to avoid anemia, a precursor to fatigue.

- **Eat breakfast.** Eating breakfast helps you start your day with a boost of energy by giving your body energy to burn. Since the brain relies on glucose for fuel, make sure to eat a breakfast that includes healthy carbohydrates such as fruit and whole grains.

- **Don't skip meals.** When you skip a meal, your blood sugar may drop sharply, intensifying fatigue. Eating regularly but modestly will help you maintain your energy levels throughout the day.

- **Avoid large meals.** Eating one or two large meals in a day can steal your energy. Blood rushes to your stomach, leaving your brain deprived and slow. Opt instead for 5 or 6 small meals to keep blood sugar and insulin levels constant.

- **Drink plenty of water.** If you're not drinking enough water, you may be dehydrated, an often overlooked cause of fatigue. Dehydration can result in reduced blood flow to organs, making you feel slow and sluggish. Aim for eight glasses of water a day; don't wait until you feel thirsty.

- **Avoid caffeine, nicotine, and other stimulants.** Caffeine may provide a temporary boost of energy when consumed moderately. However, drinking 5 or 6 caffeinated beverages per day may leave you irritable and jittery; furthermore, if you miss a caffeine fix, your fatigue will intensify. Limit your intake of coffee and sodas, and avoid caffeine completely after 6 pm, since it can touch off insomnia. Because smokers experience nicotine withdrawal symptoms at night, they can have a hard time falling asleep and awakening. Smoking itself can hasten fatigue because the carbon monoxide in cigarette smoke reduces the amount of oxygen available in the blood, lessening the amount accessible for energy production.

- **Avoid alcohol and other sedatives.** Since alcohol can interfere with sleep patterns, it is best not to drink any alcohol after dinner. Sedatives such as sleeping pills may help you sleep, but they do not treat the root cause of fatigue and may have adverse side effects that worsen fatigue in the long run.

Fatigue sufferers may also resort to overeating. Your responses to fatigue and to hunger are nearly identical: cortisol levels drop and insulin levels rise.[4] Precipitously low blood sugar levels prompt the desire for a quick sugar fix—such as a candy bar—to restore your falling energy. But boosting blood sugar in this rapid way is followed by a blood sugar crash—and intensified fatigue. Frequent eating can also slow you down, since the digestive process expends energy (think how sluggish you feel after a large meal). And as with sodas or sweetened coffee drinks, reaching for a candy bar or cookie too often can set the stage for weight gain and diabetes.

In Chapter 3, we introduce Ubiquinol, a safer and natural way to boost your body's energy supply. We describe findings on how Ubiquinol can act at the cellular level to replenish energy.

CHAPTER 2

Cardiovascular Diseases and Ubiquinol

Heart disease and stroke remain the leading causes of disability and death in America. The American Heart Association estimates that nearly 71 million US adults are afflicted with some form of cardiovascular disease.[5] It is responsible for more than 30% of all the deaths in the United States, more than all forms of cancer combined.[6] Although men generally have cardiovascular diseases at higher rates than women, that changes after women reach menopause; CVD is the leading specific cause of death for postmenopausal women, accounting for more deaths than all other causes combined.[7]

Forms of Cardiovascular Disease

- **Coronary artery disease (CAD)**[8]—In CAD, the arteries that supply blood to the heart muscle have become obstructed, most likely as a result of atherosclerosis. This may result in angina (chest pain) or myocardial infarction (heart attack), in which the heart muscle is damaged as a blood clot blocks the flow of blood through a coronary artery already nearly blocked by plaque.

- **Cardiomyopathy**[9]—Cardiomyopathy results when the heart muscle itself is diseased. Different types include ischemic, or loss of heart muscle resulting from reduced coronary blood flow; dilated, in which the heart chambers are enlarged; and hypertrophic, in which the heart muscle is thickened.

- **Congestive heart failure**[10] is a condition in which the heart muscle is weakened—as a result of CAD or cardiomyopathy, for example—and cannot pump enough blood to supply the body's organs. It may cause severe fatigue, shortness of breath, swelling in the legs and ankles, and fluid buildup in the lungs.

- **Hypertension**, or high blood pressure, occurs when blood is pumped through your vessels with excessive force (a systolic pressure of 140 mm Hg or higher and/or a diastolic pressure of 90 mm Hg or higher). High blood pressure directly increases the risk of coronary heart disease and stroke, especially along with other risk factors.[11] It is the most common form of cardiovascular disease in the Western world, affecting approximately one in three Americans.[12]

- **Stroke** occurs when a clot or rupture of a vessel interrupts blood flow to the brain, leading to brain tissue damage.[13]

Most forms of cardiovascular disease are related to common, preventable risk factors. These include diets high in saturated fat, lack of exercise, smoking, and being overweight.[14] Though each of these factors is avoidable with changes in lifestyle, relatively few Americans are making such changes. A 2005 study published in the *Archives of Internal Medicine* showed that only 3% of respondents aged 18 to 74 possessed all 4 "healthy lifestyle characteristics": not smoking, maintaining a healthy weight, eating 5 fruits and vegetables per day, and regular physical activity. Yet the benefits from lifestyle modifications are impressive. For example, in a study of individuals aged 70 to 90 a Mediterranean-style diet and greater physical activity were associated with 65%–73% lower rates of mortality associated with cardiovascular disease and cancer.[15] Other modifiable risk factors include insulin resistance and diabetes, high blood cholesterol, stress, depression, and an absence of key nutrients including omega-3 fatty acids.

Treatment Limitations

In addition to making lifestyle recommendations, doctors may recommend a variety of pharmaceutical and surgical therapies to prevent and treat the various forms of cardiovascular disease. However, all of these medical interventions carry with them the possibility of unpleasant side effects and even serious complications.

Since atherosclerosis, the buildup of plaque on the arteries, is the number one cause of cardiovascular diseases, physicians may prescribe serum cholesterol-lowering drugs known as statins. However, statins may impair normal liver function and carry the risk of muscle damage. Other side effects may include cognitive function impairment[16,17] and even rare but serious side effects such as rhabdomyolysis[18] and peripheral neuropathy.[19] These statin-related adverse effects may have even more profound implications in the elderly, due to their already-increased risk for neurodegenerative diseases and the fact that even modestly decreased cognitive and physical function in the older elderly can lead to increased disability, hospitalization, institutionalization, and mortality.[20]

It is estimated that more than 30 million Americans take statins, drugs that form a class of hyperlipidemic agents used as pharmaceuticals to lower cholesterol levels in people at risk for cardiovascular disease. Statin drugs lower cholesterol levels by inhibiting the biosynthesis of cholesterol. Statins are effective in reducing cholesterol synthesis, but not very selective as they also inhibit the biosynthesis of other important metabolites—such as coenzyme Q10 (CoQ10). Since cholesterol and CoQ10 share the same biosynthetic pathway, CoQ10 synthesis is also inhibited by statin drugs.

Statins are generally considered to be safe and effective. However, statin therapy is generally a long-term regime employed to maintain lower cholesterol levels. Many patients may develop muscle symptoms related to statin treatment.[21,22] Even in the absence of clinically relevant muscle damage, a significant number of statin users may complain of myopathic symptoms including weakness, muscle pain, cramps and fatigue.[23,24] Statin-related symptoms affect quality of life, often resulting in multiple dose alterations, switching statins, and ultimately, non-compliance. Studies show that statin-related muscle symptoms are reported by up to 10%–20% of people on statin therapy.[20,25]

It is especially important to note that people who take statins may be at even greater risk because their bodies may not convert CoQ10 to Ubiquinol efficiently and this is then compounded by the resulting lower levels of CoQ10. The heart has a very high concentration of mitochondria as it is one of the most energy-demanding organs in the body. Depletion of Ubiquinol and ubiquinone can induce mitochondrial dysfunction, critically decreasing energy production and aerobic capacity required for normal heart function.[26,27,28]

High blood pressure also sets the stage for a variety of cardiovascular conditions. Decreased plasma levels of the antioxidant CoQ10 have been observed in patients treated with statins[29] ; this can be explained by the fact that CoQ10 and cholesterol share the same biosynthetic pathway. Statins can reduce serum levels of CoQ10 by up to 40%.[30] These decreases may lead to the muscle and cognitive problems associated with statins. Chapter 3 gives a detailed explanation of the function of CoQ10 and Ubiquinol, and Chapter 4 describes evidence that CoQ10 treatment may relieve certain side effects associated with statins as well as medicines used to decrease blood pressure, including diuretics and beta blockers, which are commonly prescribed. Diuretics can decrease the body's supply of potassium, leading to muscle weakness, while beta blockers can elicit fatigue or slow heart beat. Both types of drugs can intensify the effects of diabetes. Like statins, beta blockers can also deplete levels of CoQ10.[31]

In Chapter 4, we discuss how Ubiquinol plays an essential role in cardiac health. We describe the cardiovascular benefits of Ubiquinol supplementation, compare the effects of dosing with Ubiquinol vs conventional CoQ10, and introduce findings on how Ubiquinol can provide complementary support to conventional treatments without side effects.

CHAPTER 3

Ubiquinol: Function and Benefits

WHAT IS COENZYME Q10?

Coenzyme Q10 (CoQ10) is a fat-soluble, essential quinone molecule found in nearly every cell, tissue, and organ in the body. So prevalent is CoQ10 that it was given the name ubiquinone, from the word "ubiquitous": found everywhere, and quinone. It is often called "vitamin-like" because even though it is synthesized in the membranes of human cells, it can also be acquired in small amounts from the diet; research by Kishi et al of patients receiving total parenteral nutrition without CoQ10 supplementation suggests that up to two thirds of plasma CoQ10 comes from the diet.[32] Foods with the highest concentrations of CoQ10 include dark, leafy green vegetables like broccoli and spinach, nuts, seafood, and meats, particularly organ meats: tissues with particularly high energy demands. However, even a diet rich in these foods is not adequate to offset the decline in levels of CoQ10 that occurs naturally with age. Also, since it is synthesized from the amino acid tyrosine with the aid of at least eight vitamins (vitamin C and several B-complex vitamins) and trace minerals, an insufficiency in these compounds can lead to a deficiency of CoQ10.

CoQ10 is a coenzyme, meaning that it partners with other enzymes in the body to produce particular reactions. It plays two vital roles in cellular and bodily health:

1. energy production

2. free radical protection.

HISTORY OF CoQ10[33]

CoQ10 was first discovered and isolated from beef heart mitochondria in 1957 by Dr. Fred Crane and colleagues at the University of Wisconsin.[34]At the same time, Professor R.A. Morton in England isolated the compound from vitamin A-deficient rat liver and identified it as being the same compound as CoQ10.[35] He named the compound "ubiquinone", meaning the ubiquitous quinone. Dr. Karl Folkers and his group at Merck in 1958 then identified the compound's chemical structure and were the first to produce it by fermentation. They named the compound coenzyme Q10 because of its quinone structure and the ten isoprene unit side chain.[36]

In the mid-1960's, Professor Yamamura of Japan became the first to use coenzyme Q7, a related compound, in the treatment of human disease: congestive heart failure. In 1972, Littarru and Folkers documented a deficiency of CoQ10 in human heart disease.[37,38] Dr. Peter Mitchell of England received the Nobel Prize in 1978 for his contribution to the understanding of biological energy transfer through the formulation of the chemiosmotic theory, which includes the vital protonmotive role of CoQ10 in energy transfer systems.[39] Lars Ernster of Sweden expanded upon CoQ10's importance as an antioxidant and free radical scavenger.[40]

By the mid-1970's, the Japanese perfected the industrial technology to produce pure CoQ10 in quantities sufficient for larger clinical trials. This was followed in the early 1980's by a considerable acceleration in the number and size of clinical trials, resulting in part from the availability of pure CoQ10 in large quantities from pharmaceutical companies in Japan and from the capacity to directly measure CoQ10 in blood and tissue by high performance liquid chromatography. There have now been eight international symposia on the biomedical and clinical aspects of CoQ10 from 1976 through 1993, including over 300 papers presented by approximately 200 different physicians and scientists from 18 different countries.

Professor Karl Folkers received the Priestly Medal from the American Chemical Society in 1986 and the National Medal of Science from President Bush in 1990 for his work with CoQ10 and other vitamins.

In 2006, the first pure, stable form of Ubiquinol was developed in bulk for the manufacture and commercial use of Ubiquinol as a supplement.

Man, like machine, needs a consistent supply of energy to keep running smoothly. The cells convert nutrients into an energy-rich molecule called ATP; Ubiquinol provides the spark that ignites the reaction. Structures known as "mitochondria" are the cellular equivalent of the internal combustion engine: more than 95% of the ATP in our bodies is produced in the mitochondria. Along a pathway called the electron transport chain, CoQ10 picks up electrons from one constituent of the chain, thus becoming the electron-rich, Ubiquinol form, which transfers the electrons to another constituent of the chain.[41] In this way, the electrons transfer their energy to create ATP, which provides 95% of the energy necessary for the body to carry out its various functions. Take out or significantly deplete Ubiquinol, and the machine—your body—will grind to a halt.

At the same time, the creation of ATP generates unstable molecules called free radicals. Other sources generating free radicals may include invading toxins such as cigarette smoke, pollution, and unhealthy fats. Free radicals are unstable molecules with an unpaired electron; therefore, they are looking to extract an electron from another molecule. Cellular sources for those electrons are proteins, lipids and even DNA,[42] which get damaged by this process, known as oxidation. Antioxidants help neutralize free radicals by donating an electron before the free radical damages those important cellular components. Over time, free-radical stress can give rise to a variety of disease states[43,44]; oxidation of LDL, for example, is a precursor to atherosclerosis.

The reduced form of CoQ10—Ubiquinol—is the antioxidant form, a sort of coat of armor for cells. Ubiquinol and other antioxidants give up their own electrons to neutralize the free radicals, decreasing cellular damage. In fact, Ubiquinol is one of the most potent lipophilic antioxidants, capable of regenerating other antioxidants such as tocopherol (Vitamin E) and ascorbate (Vitamin C).[45] In addition, studies show that Ubiquinol "appears to both inhibit the initiation step and interfere with the propagation step of lipid and protein oxidation, a property not apparent in the case of other antioxidants."[42]

WHAT ARE ANTIOXIDANTS?

Oxygen is life's essential element. Every time we take a breath we inhale oxygen, which drives cellular respiration and metabolism, or the creation of energy. Yet while oxygen nourishes cells, the production of energy produces a byproduct called free radicals. These are unstable molecules that lack one electron and aggressively seek a replacement from other molecules, a process called oxidation. Free radicals can be beneficial in small amounts; they perform critical metabolic functions in addition to attacking viruses and bacteria. However, at high levels they can damage important cellular components such as DNA, protein and lipids, setting the stage for a host of diseases and even premature aging.[1,2] The number of oxidative hits that occur daily to DNA per human cell is estimated at 10,000 times.[46]

Antioxidants react with free radicals before they can attack cellular components, through neutralizing their electrical charge (cancer.gov). This blocks not only the free radicals produced by metabolism but also those produced as a result of environmental insult, for example radiation, pesticides, cigarette smoke, and engine exhaust.

There are literally hundreds of naturally occurring antioxidants. While some are produced by the body, others can only be obtained through food or supplements. Brightly colored fruits and vegetables like blueberries, tomatoes, spinach, carrots, and corn, as well as drinks like green tea and red wine, are known to be rich in antioxidants. Antioxidants may take the form of vitamins, minerals, carotenoids, or polyphenols, among others. Some of the most important antioxidants found in food include vitamins A, C, and E; beta-carotene; the mineral selenium; lutein; and lycopene.[47]

Research suggests that certain key antioxidants—vitamins C and E, glutathione, lipoic acid, and Ubiquinol—may cooperate to greatly enhance each other's effects.[48] They appear to recycle, or regenerate, one another after they have neutralized a free radical, thereby extending their protective potential.[7] Furthermore, each antioxidant has a unique niche within the cell. Fat-soluble antioxidants such as vitamin E and Ubiquinol protect the fatty portion of the cell membrane, while water-soluble antioxidants such as vitamin C and glutathione shield watery portions of the cell or blood. Antioxidant-mediated free radical protection can lead to a variety of health benefits. Antioxidant reactions can affect the expression of genes; stimulate the immune response; and normalize the balance of hormone-like chemicals in the body that control pain, inflammation, and fever. Research suggests antioxidants can:

- Support the function of the aging immune system

- Decrease expression of harmful gene products and greatly reduce our risk of developing certain hereditary diseases

- Decrease age-related memory loss and mental problems

- Improve concentration and focus in people suffering from attention-deficit disorder

- Relieve symptoms of arthritis and other inflammatory conditions

- Decrease risk of heart disease and stroke

- Minimize the visible signs of aging skin and protect against skin cancer[4]

As we age, the levels of antioxidants in our bodies fall. Due to the natural course of aging and the increasing reach of environmental toxins, it may be difficult to get the optimal amount of antioxidants through food alone; dietary supplements may be of benefit to optimize and maintain a healthy cellular redox balance.

What is Ubiquinol, and what is it for?
How does it differ from the conventional oxidized form CoQ10 (ubiquinone)?

After ubiquinone, the more common form of commercially available CoQ10, is consumed, the cells immediately convert it into Ubiquinol in the cells of a healthy young person. The efficiency of this critical conversion to Ubiquinol decreases as we age, and becomes more and more compromised with oxidative stress and in various disease states. Basically, there is a small but very significant structural and functional difference between ubiquinone (the oxidized CoQ10 form) and Ubiquinol (the reduced CoQ10 form). Ubiquinol has two additional hydrogens (with the addition of two electrons) as seen on the left in the figure below.

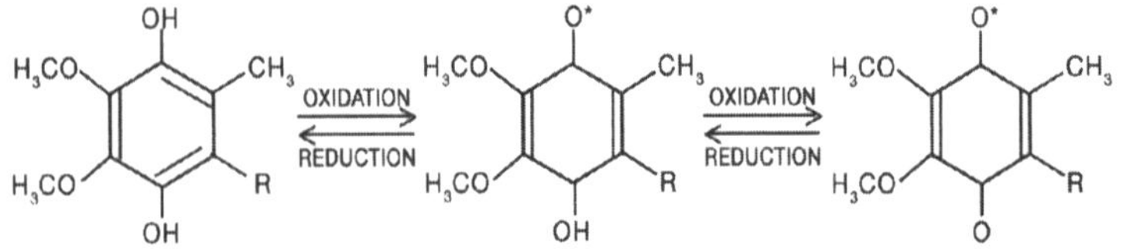

Reduced coenzyme Q10 (Ubiquinol) | Semiquinone radical $R:(CH_2CHC(CH_3)CH_2)_{10}H$ | Coenzyme Q10 (Ubiquinone)

This enzymatically driven conversion in the mitochondria facilitates the critical transfer of electrons in the mitochondrial electron transport chain, which is fundamental to subsequent ATP production. Additionally, it is the transfer of these reducing agents that confer the strong lipid-soluble active antioxidant activity of the Ubiquinol form in the mitochondria, cells, tissues and the blood. Ubiquinol is considered to be the strongest lipid soluble antioxidant that is biosynthesized, providing an active defense against oxidative insult to lipids, proteins and DNA.

In young healthy people, more than 90% of the CoQ10 in the blood exists as Ubiquinol.[49,50,51] Since the body must take an extra step in order to convert supplemental ubiquinone into Ubiquinol, full processing of ubiquinone can be metabolically challenging. As people age, their total levels of CoQ10 decline[52] and so does their ability to convert it into Ubiquinol. Some reports say this decline becomes apparent around 40 years of age, some as early as 20 with slow but continuous decline. The decrease in Ubiquinol and total CoQ10 can be due to several factors including decreasing ability of our bodies to produce (biosynthesize) adequate amounts of CoQ10, decreased conversion to Ubiquinol, an insufficiency of CoQ10 in the diet, deficiency of factors required for biosynthesis and conversion, gene mutation, oxidative insult, or the effect of various outside influences such as stress or disease. Low levels of Ubiquinol and total CoQ10 have been reported in people experiencing various disease states including (but not limited to) cardiovascular disease, neurodegenerative diseases,[53] liver disease,[54] hypertension, immunodeficiency, gingivitis, diabetes,[55] metabolic syndrome, treatment with chemotherapy and treatment with statins.[20] The result is less cellular energy, slower conversion to the reduced form and subsequently diminished protection against oxidative insult.

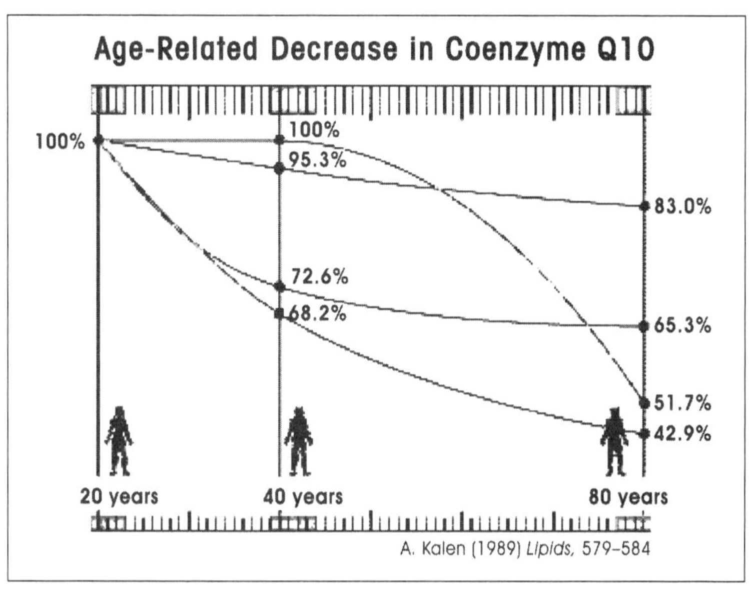

Ingesting Ubiquinol offers an easier way to replenish and maintain optimum plasma levels. However, until recently, Ubiquinol was not available in supplemental capsule form. Ubiquinol is naturally sensitive to air and light and when exposed to air undergoes auto-oxidation (loses the two extra electrons) back to ubiquinone (CoQ10), making it difficult to manufacture in bulk in a pure, stable form. Now, for the first time, scientists have successfully engineered a way to supply Ubiquinol in a pure, stable form. They established technology that enables the manufacture of Ubiquinol in bulk, and its encapsulated form, in a stable version; and have confirmed its safety in preclinical toxicity studies and published human clinical studies.[56] After the formal FDA submission for Ubiquinol as a New Dietary Ingredient, it been manufactured in the United States since 2008.

Both forms of CoQ10, ubiquinone and Ubiquinol, are redox active and play very important metabolic roles in conversion from one form to the other. Both CoQ10 forms are essential for the maintenance of energy homeostasis, cell growth, development and viability and are of specific importance in targeted areas. However, Ubiquinol is more readily absorbed in the intestinal tract and is therefore considered more "bioavailable". Studies have shown that 300 mg of Ubiquinol in a softgel can produce the same plasma level increases as 2,400 mg of ubiquinone in a chewable tablet.[56] Additionally, only the Ubiquinol form has the antioxidant capability of protecting the cells from damage due to free radicals.

Therefore, if you are young and healthy, up to the age of 30, you may meet your needs with ubiquinone, the oxidized form of CoQ10. However, if you are older (30 years and over)—a baby-boomer or beyond—and/or suffering from chronic disease or are compromised by excessive oxidative stress you may want to consider supplementation with Ubiquinol to more readily replenish this important cellular antioxidant. Ubiquinol:ubiquinone ratios have been shown to be lowered in individuals with cardiovascular, neurological, liver-related and diabetes-related[57] conditions.

Studies and Research:
The Health Benefits of Ubiquinol

THE ROLE OF ENERGY METABOLISM IN CARDIAC HEALTH

To understand the role of Ubiquinol in cardiac health, it is necessary to understand the process of energy metabolism in the heart. As we learned in Chapter 3, CoQ10 is the spark plug of energy metabolism within the cell, igniting the formation of ATP, the body's primary fuel. In the heart, ATP is used for three basic functions:

1. Contraction—to keep the heart pumping consistently

2. Relaxation—to allow the heart to rest between beats

3. Molecular synthesis—to keep the heart in good repair by building important cellular components

The energy demands of the heart are among the highest in the body. It takes energy for the ventricles of the heart to contract as they pump blood to the arteries, but it takes even more energy to relax the contracted muscle. The heart must generate ATP millions of times per second in every cell. Without enough ATP in the "energy pool," the heart's function would be compromised.

Food and oxygen are the basic building blocks of ATP creation, yet in cardiovascular disease the heart is often deprived of sufficient oxygen due to the buildup of plaque in the arteries, blocking a sufficient blood supply. The longer the deprivation, the greater the loss of its energy pool, and the harder it is for the heart to recover even after normal function is restored through medication or surgery.

THE IMPACT OF UBIQUINOL LEVELS
IN CARDIAC HEALTH

Decreased levels of Ubiquinol in patients taking cardiovascular medications such as statins[58] can impair ATP synthesis. Since Ubiquinol is so crucial in the energy metabolism process, the heart tissues of these patients may not be able to synthesize nearly enough ATP to meet their energy demands.

In addition to supporting energy production, the Ubiquinol form of CoQ10 acts as an antioxidant to protect heart cell mitochondria from free radical damage. Mitochondrial DNA is particularly vulnerable because it does not have a protective membrane. Further, Ubiquinol can limit the oxidation of LDL cholesterol[59]; inadequate availability may further contribute to atherosclerosis.

THE CARDIAC BENEFITS
OF UBIQUINOL SUPPLEMENTATION

While studies have shown that supplementation with CoQ10 can improve clinical outcomes in a number of cardiovascular diseases, not all treated patients have shown such improvement. This may have been because their plasma Ubiquinol levels did not increase sufficiently with conventional CoQ10.[60]

Ubiquinol has the potential to provide even more benefits than conventional CoQ10 because it seems to be more bioavailable and raises blood levels more significantly in these severely compromised patients. In a comparison of Ubiquinol and ubiquinone dosing (100 mg three times daily) in older healthy subjects, the plasma concentration of CoQ10 in the Ubiquinol-dosed subjects was twice that of the ubiquinone-dosed group (5.2 vs 2.5 µg/ml respectively) and the ratio of CoQ10 to cholesterol was also approximately twice as high in the Ubiquinol-dosed group (1.1 vs 0.5 µmol/mmol).

Increased benefits have been observed in several case studies. Langsjoen and Langsjoen found that a group of patients with end-stage NYHA Class IV congestive heart failure had low absorption of CoQ10 even when given doses of up to 900 mg/day of conventional CoQ10 (ubiquinone). They reported on seven of these patients who were worsening in spite of treatment with CoQ10 as well as drugs such as digitalis, diuretics, potassium, ACE inhibitors, angiotensin receptor blockers, beta blockers, nitrates, antiarrhythmics and coumadin. When these patients were then supplemented with Ubiquinol doses ranging from 150–600 mg/day, they showed an average threefold increase in plasma total CoQ10. The patients' CHF improved over periods ranging from 2–4 months, with an average twofold increase in their ejection fractions and an average improvement from NYHA Class IV to Class II in heart function. Six of the seven patients have remained stable over periods of 9–20 months on Ubiquinol. What is especially notable is the improvement in the left ventricular fraction ejection to normal range in four of the patients, which was not achieved before with the patients' previous drug and ubiquinone treatments.

TABLE 1. COQ10 LEVELS AND CHANGES IN CARDIAC FUNCTION WITH UBIQUINOL TREATMENT (from Langsjoen and Langsjoen[60])

Case	Ubiquinol Treatment (months)	Plasma CoQ10 (μg/mL)		Ejection Fraction (%)*		NYHA Class	
		Before	After	Before	After	Before	After
1	20	2.0	9.3	15	60	IV	I
2	3	0.9	2.6	35	50	IV	III
3	12	1.5	8.9	10	10	IV	III
4	10	1.7	5.1	35	60	IV	I
5	10	1.5	5.6	30	55	IV	II
6	9	2.0	5.7	10	20	IV	II
7	10	1.8	8.5	20	20	IV	III
Averages	10	1.6	6.5	22	39	IV	II

*Measurement of the capacity at which your heart is pumping; "ejection fraction" refers to the percentage of blood that's pumped out of a filled ventricle with each heartbeat. Normal is 55–70%.[61]

NEW YORK HEART ASSOCIATION (NYHA) CLASSIFICATION SYSTEM[62]	
CLASS	**PATIENT SYMPTOMS**
Class I (Mild)	No limitation of physical activity. Ordinary physical activity does not cause undue fatigue, palpitation, or dyspnea (shortness of breath).
Class II (Mild)	Slight limitation of physical activity. Comfortable at rest, but ordinary physical activity results in fatigue, palpitation, or dyspnea.
Class III (Moderate)	Marked limitation of physical activity. Comfortable at rest, but less than ordinary activity causes fatigue, palpitation, or dyspnea.
Class IV (Severe)	Unable to carry out any physical activity without discomfort. Symptoms of cardiac insufficiency at rest. If any physical activity is undertaken, discomfort is increased.

Dr. Langsjoen described a 65-year-old man with advanced ischemic cardiomyopathy on maximal medical therapy with diuretics, digitalis, beta-blocker, coumadin, and a biventricular implantable cardiac defibrillator, who required frequent admissions for Class IV congestive heart failure with severe recurrent pulmonary edema and lower extremity edema representing both right and left heart failure. In an initial evaluation (June 2006), on 450 mg of soybean oil based CoQ10, the patient's plasma CoQ10 level was sub-therapeutic at 1.6 µg/ml, and an echocardiogram on that date revealed a 15% ejection fraction with moderately severe mitral regurgitation. The patient was then changed to the Ubiquinol formulation at exactly the same dosage of 450 mg daily, and by September 2006, the plasma CoQ10 level increased to 6.4 µg/ml. An echocardiogram performed the following month showed an improvement in ejection fraction up to the 35%–40% range and a reduction in the degree of mitral regurgitation down to moderate. By this time, the patient no longer required any diuretics and his functional status was markedly improved. By January 2007, his echocardiogram showed further improvement—

up to a 45% ejection fraction—and continued clinical improvement to the point of becoming quite active, and he has required no further hospitalizations.

This cardiology group has repeated these studies, continuing to treat additional patients with end-stage or far advanced congestive heart failure with similar remarkable findings.

CHAPTER 5

The Ubiquinol Forum: Frequently Asked Questions

What is Ubiquinol?

Ubiquinol is the reduced, active antioxidant form of coenzyme Q10 (CoQ10). Produced naturally within healthy bodies, Ubiquinol is CoQ10 that has been converted (activated by the addition of two electrons) for use in the cellular energy production process. In addition to its critical role in energy production, Ubiquinol is the strongest lipid-soluble antioxidant available, protecting the body's cells from oxidative stress, which can cause damage to proteins, lipids and DNA. In young healthy individuals, Ubiquinol is the predominant form found in all tissues and cells.

What is the difference between ubiquinone and Ubiquinol?

Ubiquinone and Ubiquinol are both forms of CoQ10, and both are necessary to produce cellular energy. Ubiquinone is the oxidized form of CoQ10 with which consumers are most familiar; it has been taken as a supplement and studied for more than 30 years. Over the past three decades, CoQ10 has been recognized for its benefits to general health and wellness as well as cardiovascular and neurological health.

In order to generate cellular energy, the body needs to convert ubiquinone into Ubiquinol. Ubiquinol is the active electron transporter in the Electron Transport Chain that helps generate the energy-rich molecule ATP. Without this conversion, the body's energy production process cannot be completed and energy levels cannot be sustained. Ubiquinol, with the added electrons, (unlike the oxidized conventional CoQ10), is the powerful antioxidant that protects the cells from oxidative damage.

Why should I be concerned about declining Ubiquinol levels?

A decline in Ubiquinol decreases cellular energy and protection against oxidative stress, which produces free radicals and can damage the body's cells, including proteins, lipids and DNA. Ubiquinol provides a strong first-stage defense against this cellular oxidative damage and needs to be replenished to maintain optimum health.

An increasing number of scientific reports indicate that dramatic decreases in Ubiquinol levels and increased oxidative stress are associated with the aging process and with many age-related diseases such as cardiovascular disease, neurodegenerative disease, diabetes, cancer, fatigue and metabolic syndrome, as well as a number of other conditions.

Why does supplementing with Ubiquinol become more important as I age?

As a healthy 20-year-old, you readily produce all of the CoQ10 you can use and efficiently convert it into Ubiquinol. In fact, the predominant form of CoQ10 in the plasma, cells, tissues and organs of a healthy individual is the active Ubiquinol form.

However, age and disease impair the body's ability to produce and metabolize CoQ10. Most critical is the decline in conversion to the active Ubiquinol form. Some reasons for this include increased metabolic demand, disease, insufficient dietary intake, oxidative stress, or any combination of these factors. Some reports say this decline becomes apparent around 40 years old, although it can begin as early as 20 with slow but continuous decline. As the body's ability to produce CoQ10 and convert to Ubiquinol decreases, supplementation with Ubiquinol becomes increasingly important to maintaining optimum health.

How do I know which form of CoQ10 is right for me?

For young, healthy individuals, Ubiquinol should usually be sufficient for supplementation needs. Healthy adults in their 20s can usually convert CoQ10 into Ubiquinol; thus, supplementing with CoQ10 likely will be sufficient to raise CoQ10 levels.

For individuals who are 30+ that want to maintain an active healthy lifestyle or for those who are affected by fatigue and chronic disease, Ubiquinol is likely more beneficial since the body's ability to produce CoQ10 and convert it into Ubiquinol is diminished. Ubiquinol levels have been shown to be suppressed in individuals with cardiovascular and diabetes-related conditions. Because Ubiquinol is pre-converted, it is ready for immediate use by the body.

How much Ubiquinol should I take?

The recommended dose of Ubiquinol varies based on each individual's needs and the specific condition being treated. However, those who are older or suspect they have decreased CoQ10 due to disease may want to start supplementing with 200–300 mg of Ubiquinol per day. Studies show that the plasma levels plateau at about two weeks at this dose. Then, 100 mg per day is a good maintenance dose.

If CoQ10 has been available in supplement form for 30 years, why has Ubiquinol only recently become available?

Since Ubiquinol is easily oxidized in the air (converts back to the oxidized CoQ10 ubiquinone form), it had initially been difficult to develop a pure, active Ubiquinol form in bulk that could be made available in a supplement form. However, using advanced technology, scientists have been able to perfect a stabilization process by which Ubiquinol remains in its active electron-rich form that can still be successfully incorporated into softgel capsules.

Can I get Ubiquinol from the foods I eat?

Ubiquinol is present in some foods but is often converted to the ubiquinone form under cooking conditions. You can get Ubiquinol in small amounts from your diet; however, you would have to eat the foods in such large amounts as to make them an impractical resource for your supplementation needs. And because the body's ability to convert ubiquinone to Ubiquinol declines with age, food becomes a less practical source of Ubiquinol for older individuals and those suffering from age-related conditions.

What are the health benefits associated with Ubiquinol?

Ubiquinol provides optimal cellular energy and active antioxidant defense for a healthy active lifestyle. For those individuals who cannot efficiently convert CoQ10 to Ubiquinol, this supplement will restore healthy levels of CoQ10 in plasma and organs for more efficient energy production. This should result in more energy and stamina as well as better overall health. Additionally, because Ubiquinol is an extremely powerful antioxidant, it offers a strong protective defense against oxidative stress and age-related diseases.

If only one company makes Ubiquinol, why have I seen numerous Ubiquinol products from different companies on store shelves?

The company that manufactures Ubiquinol does not sell directly to customers; rather, it sells its ingredients to companies that make consumer supplement products. Thus, there are many brands of Ubiquinol supplements on the market today.

How long will I have to take Ubiquinol before feeling the benefits?

Not very long at all, although Ubiquinol is not a quick fix for those looking for increased energy. Unlike caffeine and other stimulants or excess sugar, which boost energy levels quickly and can cause a "crash" later, Ubiquinol offers sustained natural energy. Although it generally takes two to three weeks to restore optimal levels in blood plasma and tissues, most people will begin feeling the effects as their individual plasma levels start to increase, generally around the fifth day. Clinical studies are currently under way to determine if those affected by specific diseases may notice a decrease in the severity of their symptoms as exhibited in the study with Class 4 cardiovascular patients.

I've heard that Ubiquinol "sustains your natural energy." What does that mean?

Ubiquinol is required for the body to generate cellular energy in the form of ATP. Restoring Ubiquinol to optimal levels in people over 30 will restore the same type of youthful energy the body produced when it could efficiently convert CoQ10 to Ubiquinol and maintain adequate concentrations of Ubiquinol in plasma and tissues. Thus, supplementing with Ubiquinol is the ideal way to restore and sustain your natural energy to optimum levels.

What kind of clinical studies have been conducted on Ubiquinol?

Scientists and researchers have been studying this nutrient for more than a decade and have conducted numerous safety and toxicity studies on the ingredient. Additionally, as a form of CoQ10, Ubiquinol will have all of the same benefits of CoQ10.

In fact, since the discovery of CoQ10 there are numerous scientific studies published on Ubiquinol elucidating and further evaluating its critical role in cellular energy production and its important protective effects as the strongest know lipid soluble antioxidant.

Now that Ubiquinol has become commercially available as a supplement on a large scale scientists have had the opportunity to study the specific benefits of Ubiquinol as never before. A number of promising studies and trials are under way. Some of the various areas of immediate interest include (but are not limited to):

- Cardiovascular Disease (various forms of CVD such as Congestive Heart Failure, Statin-Induced Myalgia, Hypertension, and more)

- Huntington's Disease

- Parkinson's Disease

- Down's Syndrome

- Diabetes

- Aging

- Mitochondrial Disease

- Sports Fitness—performance, endurance and recovery

- Fatigue

Resources

For additional information on Ubiquinol, please visit:
www.ubiquinol.org/

Additional References

1. Department of Health and Human Services. Centers for Disease Prevention and Control. Chronic Fatigue Syndrome: Symptoms. Available at: www.cdc.gov/cfs/cfssymptomsHCP.htm. Accessed April 10, 2010.

2. Department of Health and Human Services. Centers for Disease Prevention and Control. Chronic Fatigue Syndrome: Basic Facts. Available at: www.cdc.gov/cfs/cfsbasicfacts.htm. Accessed April 10, 2010.

3. Reeves WC, Jones JF, Maloney E, et al. Prevalence of chronic fatigue syndrome in metropolitan, urban, and rural Georgia. *Popul Health Metr.* 2007; 5:5–14.

4. Spiegel K, Leproult R, Van Cauter E. Impact of sleep debt on metabolic and endocrine function. *Lancet.* 1999; 354(9188):1435–1439.

5. Thom T, Haase N, Rosamond W, et al. Heart disease and stroke statistics: 2006 update—a report from the American Heart Association Statistics Committee and Stroke Statistics Subcommittee [published corrections appear in Circulation. 2006;113:e696; and Circulation. 2006;114:e630]. *Circulation.* 2006;113:e85–e151.

6. American Heart Association. Cardiovascular Disease Statistics. Available at: www.americanheart.org/presenter.jhtml?identifier=4478. Accessed April 10, 2010.

7. National Center for Health Statistics. Vital Statistics of the United States. 1992. Vol 11—Mortality, Part A. Hyattsville, Md: US Dept of Health and Human Services, Public Health Service;1996. DHHS publication 96–1101.

8. National Heart Lung and Blood Institute Diseases and Conditions Index. What is Coronary Heart Disease? Available at: www.nhlbi.nih.gov/

health/dci/Diseases/Cad/CAD_WhatIs.html. Last update February 2009. Accessed April 10, 2010.

9. American Heart Association. Cardiomyopathy. Available at: www. americanheart.org/presenter.jhtml?identifier=4468. Accessed April 10, 2010.

10. American Heart Association. Congestive Heart Failure. Available at: www.americanheart.org/presenter.jhtml?identifier=4585.   Accessed April 10, 2010.

11. American Heart Association. High Blood Pressure. Available at: www.americanheart.org/presenter.jhtml?identifier=4623. Accessed April 10, 2010.

12. American Heart Association. High Blood Pressure Statistics. Available at: www.americanheart.org/presenter.jhtml?identifier=4621. Accessed April 10, 2010.

13. American Stroke Association. What is Stroke? Available at: www. strokeassociation.org/presenter.jhtml?identifier=3030066. Accessed April 10, 2010.

14. A History of the Framingham Heart Study. Framingham Heart Study: a project of the National Heart, Lung and Blood Institute and Boston University. Available at: www.framinghamheartstudy.org/about/history. html. Accessed April 10, 2010.

15. Knoops KTB, LCPGM de Groot, D Kromhout, et al. Mediterranean diet, lifestyle factors, and 10–year mortality in elderly men and women. *JAMA*. 292:1433–1439.

16. Muldoon MF, Barger SD, Ryan CM, et al. Effects of lovastatin on cognitive function and psychological well-being. *Am J Med.* 2000; 108: 538–547.

17. Muldoon MF, Ryan CM, Sereika SM, et al. Randomized trial of the effects of simvastatin on cognitive functioning in hypercholesterolemic adults. *Am J Med.* 2004; 117:823–829.

18. Chang JT, Staffa JA, Parks M, Green L. Rhabdomyolysis with HMG-CoA reductase inhibitors and gemfibrozil combination therapy. *Pharmacoepidemiol Drug Saf.* 2004;13(7):417–426.

19. Backes JM, Howard PA. Association of HMG-CoA reductase inhibitors with neuropathy. *Ann Pharmacother.* 2003;37(2):274–278.

20. Golomb BA. Implications of statin adverse effects in the elderly. *Expert Opin Drug Saf.* 2005; 4(3):389–397.

21. Phillips PS, Haas RH, Bannykh S, et al. Statin-associated myopathy with normal creatine kinase levels. *Ann Intern Med.* 2002; 137: 581–585.

22. Ballantyne CM, Corsini A, Davidson MH, et al. Risk for myopathy with statin therapy in high risk patients. *Arch Intern Med.* 2003; 163: 553–564.

23. Thompson PD, Nugent AM, Herbert PN. Statin-associated myopathy. *JAMA.* 2003; 289: 1681–1690.

24. Franc S, Dejager S, Bruckert E, Chauvenet M, Giral P, Turpin G. A comprehensive description of muscle symptoms associated with lipid-lowering drugs. *Cardiovasc Drugs Ther.* 2003; 17: 459–465.

25. Bruckert E, Hayem G, Dejager S, Yau C, Bégaud B. Mild to moderate muscular symptoms with high dosage statin therapy in hyperlipidemic patients—the PRIMO Study. *Cardiovasc Drugs Ther.* 2005; 19: 403–414.

26. De Pinieux G, Chariot P, Ammi-saïd M, et al. Lipid lowering drugs and mitochondrial function: effects of HMG-CoA reductase inhibitors on serum ubiquinone and blood lactate/pyruvate ratio. *Br J Clin Pharmacol.* 1996; 42: 333–337.

27. Mabuchi H, Higashikata T, Kawashiri M, et al. Reduction of serum ubiquinol and ubiquinone levels by atorvastatin in hypercholesterolemic patients. *J Atheroscler Thromb.* 2005; 12: 111–119.

28. Caso G, Kelly P, McNurlan MA, Lawson WE. Effect of coenzyme Q10 on myopathic symptoms in patients treated with statins. *Am J Cardiol.* 2007; 99: 1409–1412.

29. Passi S, Stancato A, Aleo E, Dmitrieva A, Littarru GP. Statins lower plasma and lymphocyte ubiquinol/ubiquinone without affecting other antioxidants and PUFA. *Biofactors.* 2003;18(1–4):113–124.

30. Ghirlanda G, Oradei A, Manto A, et al. Evidence of plasma CoQ10–lowering effect by HMG-CoA reductase inhibitors: a double-blind, placebo-controlled study. *J Clin Pharmacol.* 1993;33(3): 226–229.

31. Kishi T, Watanabe T, Folkers K. Bioenergetics in clinical medicine XV. Inhibition of coenzyme Q10–enzymes by clinically used adrenergic blockers of beta-receptors. *Res Commun Chem Pathol Pharmacol.* 1977;17 (1): 157–164.

32. Kishi T, Okamoto T, Kishi H, Okada A. Serum levels of coenzyme Q10 in patients receiving total parenteral nutrition and relationship of serum lipids. In: Folkers K. and Yamamura Y. (Herausgeber) *Biomedical and Clinical Aspects of Coenzyme Q.* 1986; 5:119.

33. Adapted from: Langsjoen PH. Introduction to Coenzyme Q10. Available at: http://faculty.washington.edu/ely/coenzq10.html. Accessed April 10, 2010.

34. Crane FL, Hatefi Y, Lester RI, Widmer C. Isolation of a quinone from beef heart mitochondria. *Biochim Biophys Acta.* 1957;25:220–221.

35. Morton RA, Wilson GM, Lowe JS, Leat WMF. Ubiquinone. In: *Chemical Industry.* 1957, pp. 1649.

36. Wolf DE, Hoffman CH, Trenner NR, et al. Structure studies on the coenzyme Q group. *J Am Chem Soc.* 1958. 80:4752.

37. Littarru GP, Ho L, Folkers K. Deficiency of coenzyme Q10 in human heart disease. Part I. *Int J Vitam Nutr Res.* 1972; 42(2) 291–305.

38. Littarru GP, Ho L, Folkers K. Deficiency of coenzyme Q10 in human heart disease. Part II. *Int J Vitam Nutr Res.* 1972; 42 (3):413–434.

39. Mitchell P. The vital protonmotive role of coenzyme Q. In: Folkers K., Littarru GP, Yamagami T. (eds) *Biomedical and Clinical Aspects of Coenzyme Q, vol. 6.* Elsevier, Amsterdam, 1991, pp 3–10.

40. Ernster L. Facts and ideas about the function of coenzyme Q10 in the mitochondria. In: Folkers K., Yamamura Y. (eds) *Biomedical and Clinical Aspects of Coenzyme Q.* Elsevier, Amsterdam, 1977, pp 15–18.

41. Crane FL, Navas P. The diversity of coenzyme Q function. *Mol Aspects Med.* 1997;18:s1–s6.

42. Bentinger M, Brismar K, Dallner G. The antioxidant role of coenzyme Q. Mitochondrion 2007;7S:S41–S50.

43. Florence TM. The role of free radicals in disease. *Aust N Z J Ophthalmol.* 1995 Feb;23(1):3–7

44. Stohs SJ.The role of free radicals in toxicity and disease. *J Basic Clin Physiol Pharmacol.* 1995;6(3–4):205–28. Review.

45. Arroyo A, Navarro F, Gómez-Díaz C, et al. Interactions between ascorbyl free radical and coenzyme Q at the plasma membrane. *J Bioenerg Biomembr.* 2000;32(2):199–210.

46. Packer L, Cadenas E. Oxidants and antioxidants revisited. New concepts of oxidative stress. *Free Radic Res.* 2007;41(9):951–952.

47. Sies H, Stahl W, Sundquist AR. Antioxidant functions of vitamins. Vitamins E and C, beta-carotene, and other carotenoids. *Ann N Y Acad Sci.* 1992;669:7–20.

48. Podda M, Grundmann-Kollmann M. Low molecular weight antioxidants and their role in skin ageing. *Clin Exp Dermatol.* 2001 26: 578–582.

49. Aberg F, Appelkvist EL, Dallner G, Ernster L. Distribution and redox state of ubiquinones in rat and human tissues. *Arch Biochem Biophys.* 1992;295(2):230–234.

50. Miles MV, Horn PS, Morrison JA, Tang PH, DeGrauw T, Pesce AJ. Plasma coenzyme Q10 reference intervals, but not redox status, are affected by gender and race in self-reported healthy adults. *Clin Chim Acta.* 2003; 332(1–2):123–132.

51. Okamoto T, Matsuya T, Fukunaga Y, Kishi T, Yamagami T. Human serum ubiquinol-10 levels and relationship to serum lipids. *Int J Vitam Nutr Res.* 1989;59: 288–292.

52. Kalén A, Appelkvist EL, Dallner G. Age-related changes in the lipid compositions of rat and human tissues. *Lipids.* 1989;24:579–584.

53. Sohmiya M, Tanaka M, Suzuki Y, Tanino Y, Okamoto K, Yamamoto Y. An increase of oxidized coenzyme Q-10 occurs in the plasma of sporadic ALS patients. *J Neurol Sci.* 2005;228(1):49–53.

54. Yamamoto Y, Yamashita S. Plasma ubiquinone to ubiquinol ratio in patients with hepatitis, cirrhosis, and hepatoma, and in patients treated with percutaneous transluminal coronary reperfusion. *BioFactors.* 1999;9:241–246.

55. Lim SC, Ong CH, Trisse G, Subramaniam T, Sum CF. Mitochondrial oxidative burden in pre-diabetic and diabetic individuals—indirect evidence from plasma coenzyme Q. Presented at the 65th Scientific Sessions

of the American Diabetes Association, June 10–14, 2005, San Diego, CA, USA. (Abstract 657–P)

56. Hosoe K, Kitano M, Kishida H, Kubo H, Fujii K, Kitahara M. Study of safety and bioavailability of ubiquinol after single and 4–week multiple oral administration to healthy volunteers. *Regulatory Toxicology and Pharmacology.* 2007;47:19–28.

57. Hasegawa G, Yamamoto Y, Zhi JG, et al. Daily profile of plasma %CoQ10 level, a biomarker of oxidative stress, in patients with diabetes manifesting postprandial hyperglycemia. *Acta Diabetol.* 2005;42:179–181.

58. Folkers K, Langsjoen P, Willis R, et al. Lovastatin decreases coenzyme Q levels in humans. *Proc Natl Acad Sci USA.* 1990;87(22):8931–8934.

59. Thomas SR, Neuzil J, Stocker R. Cosupplementation with coenzyme Q prevents the prooxidant effect of alpha-tocopherol and increases the resistance of LDL to transition metal-dependent oxidation initiation. *Arterioscler Thromb Vasc Biol.* 1996;16(5):687–696.

60. Langsjoen PH, Langsjoen AM. Supplemental ubiquinol in patients with advanced congestive heart failure. *BioFactors* .2008;32:119–128.

61. Grogan M. Ejection fraction: what does it measure? MayoClinic.com. September 19, 2008. Available at www.mayoclinic.com/health/ejection-fraction/AN00360. Accessed April 10, 2010.

62. The Stages of Heart Failure—NYHA Classification. Heart Failure Society of America. Last update 2002. Available at www.abouthf.org/questions_stages.htm. Accessed April 10, 2010.

Index

About the Author

Robert J. Barry, Ph.D, focuses on clinical research development and collaboration and on the development of the technical, business and commercial translation of products and technology.

Dr. Barry was a Principal Advisor for NIH, specializing in the commercial development of biotech start-up companies and their technologies and products. He also founded and served as president of a premier independent testing laboratory and scientific research company serving the natural products industry. Prior to that, Dr. Barry developed a natural products division for a major analytical device company where he served as vice president and chief technical officer.

Dr. Barry brings more than 18 years of strategic technical development and commercial translation of scientific products, analytical services, drug development and pre-clinical evaluation systems to his position. Before that, he co-founded and served as the president of a Massachusetts-based drug development company. Under Dr. Barry's direction, the company identified new lead-drug candidates focusing on unmet clinical needs in several disease areas.

Dr. Barry earned his bachelor's degree in biology from Boston College; his Ph.D. in chemistry/biochemistry from the University of Maryland; carried out postdoctoral research in Biological Chemistry and Molecular Pharmacology at Harvard Medical School; and was a staff researcher in neuropathology at Harvard Medical School.

He is an active member of numerous professional associations including the American Chemical Society and the American Association for the Advancement of Science.